SENSORY DEPRIVATION

FLOAT TANK FOR STRESS, ANXIETY, RELAXATION, PAIN & CONSCIOUSNESS

COLE CAMPBELL

© 2016

COPYRIGHT NOTICE

All rights reserved.

No part of this publication may be reproduced, distributed, or transmitted in any form or by any means; including, photocopying, recording, or other electronic or mechanical methods, without the prior written permission of the publisher, except in the case of brief quotations embodied in critical reviews and certain other non-commercial uses permitted by copyright law.

DISCLAIMER

Although the author and publisher have made every effort to ensure that the information in this book was correct at press time, the author and publisher do not assume and hereby disclaim any liability to any party for any loss, damage, or disruption caused by errors or omissions, whether such errors or omissions result from negligence, accident, or any other cause.

This book is not intended as a substitute for the medical advice of physicians. The reader should regularly consult a physician in matters relating to his/her health and particularly with respect to any symptoms that may require diagnosis or medical attention.

Table of Contents

COPYRIGHT NOTICE ii

DISCLAIMER iii

INTRODUCTION 1

SENSORY OVERLOAD IN THE MODERN WORLD 6

EXPERIENCING SENSORY DEPRIVATION
TREATMENT 15

SENSORY INTELLIGENCE 24

THEORIES REGARDING THE BENEFITS 30

TIPS TO HELP YOU RELAX AND PREPARE FOR THE
FLOAT TANK 36

CONCLUSION 42

INTRODUCTION

The term sensory deprivation is literally the removal of one or more of your five senses. Although it has become popular in recent years for helping cope with stress and relaxing the mind and body; it is not a new idea. In fact sensory deprivation has been around in one form or another for s long as mankind has. In its most basic form it is being blindfolded, or wearing earmuffs. This will effectively remove or seriously reduce your ability to see, hear, or do either. It is possible to undertake this type of sensory deprivation as part of a sexual experience, a trust exercise or even as part of a torture technique.

There are more complicated techniques which can be used to remove heat perception, touch, taste and even gravity! It is believed that sensory deprivation in the short term can lead to a heightened sense of well being and aid in the ability to relax as well as meditate. Long term sensory deprivation has the potential to cause anxiety, depression and even hallucinations; both short term and long term issues will be looked at in more detail later in this book.

It is also worth noting that a technique known as perceptual deprivation has been used, especially by those attempting to torture others. Instead of removing one of your senses the technique can feed a specific sense uniformly and consistently. For example, the sound of water dripping into a bucket can be soothing at first but will become annoying if it continues for an extended period of time. Surprisingly this technique can also be used for short periods of time to achieve the same effect as sensory deprivation. Again, for longer periods of time it can cause negative side effects. In fact, there are five sensory deprivation techniques which were used by the British security forces in Northern Ireland; these methods have all since been declared as inhumane, as such they are no longer used:

1. Wall standing – as its name suggests this technique involves someone stood facing a wall for an extended period of time. The most effective way was to put the body into a stress position; such as head against the wall with their hands high above their head and their legs spread, with feet stepped back from the wall. The weight of the body is forced onto the toes and the fingers. Sensory deprivation occurs as they are blindfolded and lose awareness of their surroundings.
2. Hooding – refers to the technique of placing a black bag over someone's head and keeping it there for an extended period of time. The ability to see is removed, hearing seriously muffled and there is a natural response to panic.
3. Noise – Putting someone in a room with a constant hissing, or dripping noise. This is an example of perceptual deprivation as opposed to sensory deprivation although the result has been seen to be the same.
4. Sleep deprivation – As its name suggests, simply depriving someone of the opportunity to sleep.
5. Reduced Food Intake – Simply limiting food intake or preventing it altogether.

Sensory deprivation is now associated as an aid to improve your mental and physical health. It is possible to undertake it through several different methods, although the most popular currently is the Restricted Environmental stimulation Therapy (REST for short). There are actually two different ways of experiencing REST:

- Chamber REST

This is the less claustrophobic example of sensory deprivation. It must take place in a special room which has been sound proofed to either dramatically reduced or eliminate sounds from outside of the room. You enter the room and get comfortable on the bed. The session then starts and the room is placed in complete darkness. A session can last for one hour or up to twenty four. Obviously longer sessions will have breaks for refreshments and the opportunity to use the toilet. There is no physical restraint keeping you in the room, except for your personal motivation.

- Flotation REST

This option will place you in a pool of skin temperature water and Epsom salts. The pool is designed to allow you to float safely, without any health risk. Sessions usually last for about an hour and it had been shown to reduce pain, stress, and even lower blood pressure. People who have experienced the flotation tank have reported feeling itchy in various places across their body's for the first forty minutes. This has also been associated with the early stages of meditation. The last twenty minutes of an hour session are usually when your brain will switch from beta or alpha brainwaves and start producing theta. These are the brainwaves which usually happen just before falling asleep and in the first few moments of waking up. When connected with sleeping the theta brainwaves last just a few seconds, however when you are undergoing flotation REST it can last for several minutes. It is often thought that this is the most beneficial time to solve creative issues and other problems.

The original Floatation REST was a light, soundproof tank created by John C. Lilly in 1954. It was designed to monitor the effects of sensory deprivation. Unfortunately, the results are of little benefit as John C. Lilly completed his tests while taking the drug LSD. His plan was to study the brain and the amount of activity it undertakes. There has always been a question surrounding where the brain gets its energy from and John C. Lilly believed that if the stimuli were removed then the brain would resort to sleeping; it would have nothing further to do. In order to fully disconnect from reality Lilly decided that LSD would be a viable option, his studies focused on the origin of consciousness.

The first isolation tanks were uncomfortable; they required people to wear heavy breathing gear and tight clothing. They were then submerged in water although the experience was marred by the uncomfortable feel of their clothing and the weight of the oxygen tanks. This prevented many people from feeling the real isolation experience as their focus was on the fear of drowning. In the 1970's two scientists from the University of British Columbia started to explore potential therapeutic benefits from the tanks. These were the scientists who originally came up with the REST tag. Modern isolation tanks use the water and Epsom salt mix which allows you to float in the water with your ears submerged to reduce external sounds. People are encouraged to allow their arms to float away from their body and the feeling of being completely at one with the pond will gradually extend the boundary of the body; or remove it altogether.

Modern tanks are generally made of plastic and must adhere to strict build standards as well as a strict regime of cleaning chemicals. The flotation ranks have become very popular as ways to help people relax and recuperate. In contrast the chamber REST method is an extension of research that was originally started in the 1950' and has still not been completed.

Sensory deprivation has been designed to help people become more in touch with their own bodies. However, it has also proved to be an effective way of helping someone to stop smoking; treatment by itself was effective at stopping twenty five percent of smokers, treatment combined with behavioural modification resulted in a fifty percent stoppage rate and those who also had group therapy achieved an impressive eighty percent stoppage rate. This type of treatment has also been shown to be effective at helping those with alcohol and drug issues.

Entering a sensory tank is a unique experience. There is no sound, no light and no outside disturbances. You will feel and hear every creak and ache in your body as you settle into one of the most peculiar sensations of your life. The water is kept at the same temperature as your skin, which makes it very difficult to know where your body finishes and the tank begins. It is this sensation that will encourage you to push the boundaries of your mind and is probably the reason that most users report out of body experiences and even hallucinations.

Of course, every person's experience is different; it is unique to them, their personal situation and what is going on in the world around them. The experience is likely to be beneficial for a host of reasons which will be discussed in this book.

The sensory deprivation tank may have been first envisioned sixty five years ago, but it is enjoying a surge of popularity in the current market and offers the potential to help you reduce stress, anxiety and even pain. The effects of this treatment method will be discussed fully in this book along with the benefits and reasons for you to sample sensory deprivation for yourself. There is also additional information on the types of sensory deprivation and the best places to locate a sensory tank near you.

SENSORY OVERLOAD IN THE MODERN WORLD

There is no doubt that most people live incredibly hectic and stressful lives. Modern technology has invaded every part of our lives and many people are no longer able to switch off fully from their work or social commitments. Email, social media and the cloud mean that you are always connected to the various parts of your life. As much as this is often seen as a good thing, there is also a case to be made that there is no opportunity to pause and enjoy some alone time. Quite simply, people no longer have the chance to step back and see where they are going or their part in the world around them; it can be too complicated just to take a moment to stop and reflect on the world around you.

Sensory overload is a phrase that is often talked about and it may be associated with a variety of issues, although it is not always fully understood. In fact, sensory overload can apply to any situation where you are struggling to cope with all the different pressures and demands of life. It can refer to one specific area of your life or can even be a reaction to all the different elements becoming too much for you; this is often recognised as the point of a nervous breakdown.

Of course, there are many factors of life which are simply necessary to be dealt with, and it is not plausible, or even possible to ignore or bypass these factors. It is also not desirable as the majority of humans need to feel that they are part of something bigger than themselves, that they are connected to the rest of the world.

The main senses are touch, sight, hearing, taste and smell; these senses develop naturally as you grow from child into an adult. It is essential for everyone to be exposed to a variety of stimuli which will help your senses mature. As a child it is unlikely that you will experience sensory overload; this has been associated with the ability of most children to tune out unwanted or unneeded noise and information. Children can generally choose to focus on one item; they can ignore everything else going on. Research suggests that this is, in part, connected with the lack of other stresses on the body. As you age you are constantly submerged in situations which require your input and you are the one responsible for making the right decision. The main problem with this is that you are constantly dwelling on the decision and which choice to make, you are also likely to be second guessing yourself, even after the decision has been made. If you add this stress to factors such as overcrowding, urbanization and even the mass social media exposure and you will quickly have the relevant factors to cause a sensory overload.

In fact, sensory overload is something that happens to everyone for short periods of time; when everything just feels like it is on top of you. The usual solution is to simply take a few moments to breathe or focus on a different problem. Whenever possible it is worth taking five minutes to yourself to clear your mind and place the issues in perspective. There is often a tendency to feel like the world is falling apart and to react badly as no one else seems to understand the issue. However, in reality, the issue may not be as bad as it seems, it is simply that it has consumed your thoughts and senses, effectively overloading your system.

Although sensory overload has been a possibility since the first humans existed on the planet, it is only in the last twenty to thirty years that research and studies have been undertaken in an attempt to understand the human better. Georg Simmel researched and wrote one of the earliest studies in the 1990's; his theory was that urbanization is one of the major contributory factors to overstimulation of the brain, as well as the body. The Japanese followed up on this work by subjecting a select group of people to be subjected to intense and excessive audio and visual stimuli, in effect, the study looked at perceptual deprivation and its effect on sensory overload. All the subjects in the research project, appeared to have a visible mood shift; becoming more anxious, aggressive and even sad.

The results of this study by the Tohuku University in Japan led to further studies being commissioned. It became clear that submitting people to either perceptual deprivation or sensory deprivation was an initial step towards sensory overload. The majority of those who were monitored displayed a range of symptoms:

- Irritable or easily irritated by the smallest of issues.

- Overexcitement by the events going on around them, this often leads to a nervous, hyperactive approach to all and any task.

- Many of the research subjects actually started to withdraw into themselves and avoid bright lights as they became over stimulated.

The above symptoms are generally expected as someone becomes over stimulated, the following effect were also commonly witnessed but can also be linked with a variety of other disorders:

- A lack of concentration, despite the pressure placed on someone to meet targets, deadlines or perform. Sensory overload actually makes it difficult to focus for any period of time on one activity.

- This lack of concentration can be seen in an inability to relax the muscles, resulting in restlessness and fidgeting. In turn this can be exceptionally tiring and lead to sleeplessness, fatigue and even angry outbursts.

Many of these symptoms are displayed by people who are suffering from General Anxiety Disorder, there continues to be research undertaken into the connection between the two conditions.

It is important to note that sensory overload is not just an issue regarding an overly stressful working environment. It can be caused, or triggered by bright lights, fast action scenes on the television, multiple sounds at the same time (such as music, children and a discussion on politics!). It has also been linked with spicy food, a rapid change in the environment around you strong smells and even prolonged tense situations; at home or at work.

Unfortunately there are a host of side effects which can arise from sensory overload; it can lead to a reduction in your self esteem, or make you social anxious every time you need to go out; in fact extreme cases may be linked with the inability to leave your own house. In effect, your senses have become so overloaded that you wish to avoid all other interactions in order to protect your own sense of self.

The more you consider the influences on your own life the more you will become aware that most people are constantly be subjected to things which could cause a sensory overload. There is a need for balance between being busy, socially interactive and constantly existing at a hyper speed and the possibility that you will overload your senses and this can lead to health issues.

The reality is that most people live their lives at a frantic pace; the utopian future envisioned not so long ago is actually further away than ever before. Time has now become one of the most precious commodities; there is never enough of it and this is why you end up feeling overwhelmed and your sense are pushed to their limit. Unfortunately this is not just detrimental to your physical health; it can affect your mental health and leave you questioning your place in the world around you as well as your ability to cope. The feelings of being overwhelmed can often lead to depression, which, once it has taken hold, can be very difficult to escape from.

Perhaps the biggest and most difficult part of sensory overload is that it is incredibly difficult to know when someone is at risk of being over stimulated. Some people dislike entering places that they have never been into before, whilst others think nothing of it. Schools, work environments and even public transport systems can be full of loud noises and people dashing in all directions; to some this is part of the fun of life; to others, it is a sensory overload which they endure on a daily basis. As it is not possible to predict who will respond in a particular way it becomes very difficult to know who is more likely to suffer from sensory overload.

The focus must then be on dealing with sensory overload as effectively and discreetly as possible. The premise that many people live by is to work hard and play hard, this philosophy can be applied to sensory overload. The more you feel you are at risk of being overloaded the more important it will be to find a release. There are several options:

The Complete Break

Most people try to take a holiday every year, but this does not mean that they are taking a break from the sensory experiences they have every day. Not only is it possible for work to contact you via a cell phone, email or messaging service, it is also common for people to log into their work, even when on holiday!

To combat this, your annual holiday, or even a regular weekend break, should remove you from all outside influences completely. Your phone, internet access and computer should be discarded as you undertake something different to your normal daily activities. This could be working on a farm for the weekend, helping children in a third world country or simply turning off all your electronic gadgets and keeping them off for the entire weekend. At first this may actually increase the feelings associated with sensory overload as you panic over having your connection with the outside world cut. However, once you have experienced it you will become aware of a whole host of sights and sounds, particularly those of nature, which you may have forgotten existed. The feelings and experiences associated with this will immediately relieve your sensory overload and help you to keep things in perspective.

Sensory Deprivation Treatment

Most people do not have the time and, quite possibly, are literally unable to separate themselves completely from their life for a week or more. This is especially true if you have children. Although they are an incredible gift they can also contribute to the amount of stress you are under; effectively increasing your risk of sensory overload. There are a variety of treatment options available:

- Isolation – It is possible to isolate yourself completely from the rest of the world but this is not an idea way to live! There is also no guarantee that this will prevent sensory overload in the long term. Isolation actually refers to locating the source of your sensory overload and either reducing it or eliminating it from your life. Of course, there are many reasons and occasions why it may not be possible to eliminate something from your life. However, it should still be possible to reduce it or look at ways of changing the stimulus over time.

Much of this approach relies on being able to work out what triggers your sensory overload, is it the fear of heights? Or perhaps crowds? It may simply be too much of a particular food; the range of triggers is limitless! Although it may take you some time to work out which specific thing or things, is triggering your overload, it is a worthwhile exercise. Once you know you can either avoid the situation or prepare yourself mentally for it. The best way to prepare is to relax mentally and physically; you know what you will have to deal with and can be ready for it.

- Float Tank – This has already been mentioned. A tank filled with water and Epsom salts is kept at the same temperature as your body. You will float in the water and can choose to have the lid on or off. With the lid on it will be completely dark, your ears will be submerged as you float on your back and even your sense of touch will diminish as you relax and your body struggles to define where you end and the water begins.

A float tank provides you with the opportunity to remove yourself from all the stresses and strains of life for a short while. It does not change the stress you are under but it does allow you to clear your mind. The float tank does offer a variety of other benefits which are looked at later in this book.

- Isolation Room – This is similar in concept to the float tank, however, instead of being suspended, weightless in water you are confined to one room.

The room is dark and you simply lay in the bed, losing yourself within your own mind. This is an option for those who are unable to deal with the small confined space of a float tank. It is more difficult to lose your sense of touch in this environment and merge with your surroundings as, even if the room is the same temperature as your body, you will be in constant touch with the bed and gravity will have an effect.

Sensory Intelligence

This is a complicated field which requires the assistance of a therapist to help you understand the sensory implications of your actions and how you can control the sensory responses. It is a relatively new field but has been shown to have positive results for a variety of conditions and issues which are faced by everyone in the modern world. This option is discussed in more detail later in the book.

There is no doubt that the stress of modern life is a key contributor to sensory overload and that there are several options which can be utilized to help combat the issue. However, as with everything, the best solution may be a mixture of all the solutions listed in this book, or it may even be something you have devised yourself. There is no right or wrong method of treatment. It is simply important to find something that works for you and allows you to live a healthy, balanced life.

Perhaps the most important advice you can receive to help deal with sensory overload is to learn your own limits. Once you know how far you can go before you reach the point of overload you will be able to devise a phrase that stops others from continuing. Alternatively you can simply walk away from the situation. Knowing your limits and your triggers will allow you to regain control of your life almost instantly. You will then be able to work on other techniques, such as sensory deprivation, to assist you in coping with these issues in the future. It is possible to gradually stretch your tolerances. Whatever your current situation there is a way to both deal with it and improve it!

EXPERIENCING SENSORY DEPRIVATION TREATMENT

The idea of floating in warm water, whilst enclosed in a relatively small box may lead to you conjuring images of new age festivals. This image will be backed up by the fact that many people who experience this sensation report to have experienced hallucinations or out of body experiences. Indeed, John C. Lilly first invented the sensory deprivation tank simply to help him achieve out of body experiences. In fact, he is reported to have said that he had been able to contact alien life forms through the deprivation tank as his spirit lifted to another dimension. Of course, he was also using LSD; a highly hallucinogenic drug which may have influenced his results!

In reality, depriving yourself of your senses is a particularly weird sensation and you will spend the majority of your first sessions getting comfortable and used to the idea. Although people have likened it to returning to the womb, this is only really in a conceptual way as it is simply not possible to remember what it was like inside the womb! There is no doubt that the deprivation of your senses will allow your mind to slowly clear. As with any quiet time you will start by processing the thoughts and actions of the day, but as your mind quietens you are likely to find that you start considering the balance of your life and what is really important. It is at this point you are likely to struggle to distinguish where your body ends and the water begins. Unfortunately, the session is usually only an hour long and you will not spend an extended period of time in this, almost dreamlike, state. The general consensus of those who have experienced sensory deprivation is that you will emerge feeling very relaxed; it will take a short while for your body to return to normal and then you will feel better focused on what is important. Most people also sleep much better that night, either going to bed earlier or sleeping in, past their usual wake-up call; the sleep is also deeper and more fulfilling. The usual response is to have an almost supercharged burst of energy the following day!

Sensory deprivation float tanks are started to appear in a multitude of places, in fact; it is highly likely that there is one within a short drive of your house! A short search of the internet for 'float tanks' will quickly point you in the right direction. For those that have experienced these tanks on several occasions it is even possible to have a float tank fitted at home.

As with any facility it is important to confirm their standards and their costs. All float centres should be able to advise you which products they use to maintain the cleanliness of their tanks. UV and hydrogen peroxide are commonly used and offer a hygienic experience; the water should also be changed regularly, ideally every six months. The cost of the float tanks should be comparable; if it is too cheap then you will need to consider where they may be cutting corners! Finally, it is also important to consider the facilities they offer. Ideally you will be looking for a private room with shower facilities and maybe even a hairdryer. This will ensure your belongings are safe while you float and the privacy you will need afterwards is there.

There are no special requirements which you need to adhere to before entering the tank; a shower is necessary, just to remove any excess personal chemicals; deodorant, etc.

Having decided to take the plunge and experience the float tank you will be likely to experience the following thoughts and feelings:

- A feeling or fear and maybe even some excitement as you climb into your tank. This is especially true in the first occasion as you are going into an environment which is not natural for the human body. You are used to relying on your senses to know what is happening around you. A float tank will remove those senses and leave you isolated. Additionally, for the macabre, it can feel like you are closing yourself into a watery tomb!

- Many people report that it is difficult to become comfortable, you may feel itchy at first as your skin settles into the water. Although you are effectively weightless it can be difficult to find the most comfortable position. Part of this has actually been attributed to your body finding its balance and your lack of ability to orientate yourself; you may feel like you are moving or rotating when you are actually not!

- Once you have finally settled you will, undoubtedly, spend the first part of your session considering your standard issues, list of things to do, or even how you could have done something better. In the first uses of this tank you are likely to spend much of your session considering these issues.

- It is then quite common to experience a calming of your mind. You gradually stop thinking about the day to day matters and your mind is quite likely to clear completely. This is the time you are most likely to see psychedelic images. These images are more likely to be swirling patterns of colours than a clear image of anything. Some people have reported experiencing a friend or loved one in the tank with them but it is difficult to say if this is your mind focusing on a variety of abstract images and conjuring them up for you or if it is something more spiritual.

- Most people who try a float tank will comment that their time, whether an hour or two, simply disappeared and they are not quite sure whether they fell asleep, meditated or that the time just disappeared incredibly quickly.

- The best facilities have an electronic timer which will tell you that you session is over. You can then take a few moments to adjust yourself to the lightness of the room and enjoy a shower; this is essential to wash the salt of your body. You will be surprised at how soft your skin feels!

- To finish your session it is best to enjoy a cup of herbal tea and allow your body to effectively adapt back to the normal world. An hour floating in the dark can have quite an effect on your orientation and perception!

The majority of people who undertake a float session would say they have more energy and enthusiasm for life for several days afterwards.

The experience of floating weightless has also been linked with a variety of health benefits:

- Stress

Stress is a factor of everyone's life, there is always something that will ensure you concern and worry as well as potential issues at work, with the family or financially. It is this which raises the stress levels in your body and forces your body to go into fight or flight mode. The consequence of this is an elevated cortisol level as well as higher blood pressure and excess adrenaline pumping through your system. In times of need this is the right response, however, if this is happening to often it will have a detrimental effect on your body.

Anything which allows your mind to relax will help to alleviate the stress of the day and the events taking place in your life. However, the float tank is particularly effective as it can place you into a meditative state without the need to learn how to meditate! This will help you relax and see each issue for what it really is. Pausing and looking at the bigger picture will allow you to assess what is really important and take a more relaxed approach to everything else.

- Anxiety

There are many reasons to be anxious in life; these may be for similar reasons as to why you will be stressed, it may also be for a whole host of other reasons including past experiences. Post Traumatic Stress Disorder is often a result of extreme situations where your anxiety levels are exceptionally high and you are unable to process the events you have witnessed. Whatever the reason, anxiety can have a seriously detrimental effect on your life within a short space of time. You may be anxious about certain situations or you may be anxious about everything. It is quite possible that an extreme case of anxiety can prevent you from even leaving the house.

Anxiety can be very difficult to deal with as it requires you to analyse the reasons for the anxiety and then attempt to resolve these issues. It usually takes extensive amounts of therapy and, even then, there are no guarantees as to the success of the process. It is not known exactly why the float tank can help people with anxiety but there are many examples of people with extreme cases of anxiety feeling much better after just one or two sessions in a sensory deprivation tank. Research is taking place as to why this effect is possible and whether float tanks can offer other, currently unknown benefits.

- Relaxation

Soaking in a bath for half an hour will leave you feeling relaxed, floating in a tank of water, without any other distractions to any of your senses will leave you with a much deeper sense of relaxation. You are likely to feel like you have the ability to do anything after you have completed your session.

The feeling stems from two factors;

1. The first one is the water supports your body and allows every part of you to truly relax. Muscles which are always used, even when sitting, or lying down, will actually have the opportunity to relax. Your body will then feel more relaxed than you have ever known it to before! This is likely to make you feel a little heavy and disorientated when you first leave the tank, but, the feeling will quickly pass as your recharged body adjusts and is ready to tackle anything.
2. The second factor is that, after your floating session, your mind will be relaxed. It may take most of the session for your brain to stop chattering away to itself, but, you will eventually reach a stage where you have managed to completely empty your mind. This is the key to a deep relaxation and peace of mind. Being completely relaxed will allow you to refocus your thoughts and your energy on your next task whilst feeling as relaxed and ready as though you have just had the best night's sleep ever!

- Pain Relief

Float tanks were originally designed to allow your mind to be free to explore your own limits and a multitude of other dimensions. In many senses it was the dream of connecting with a higher state of consciousness and learning about other life forms. A side effect of floating weightless is that your body will relax; muscles and tendons which are constantly contracted will actually have the chance to unwind. You will become aware of aches and pains that you did not know you had! Relaxing and removing the weight from your body has always been one of the most effective ways at reducing the stress your body is under and alleviating pain. The float tank provides the perfect setting to allow your body to do this whilst your mind is expanding its awareness.

In fact, professional athletes are becoming aware of the potential of these float tanks and several of them have already started to use them to help with healing and mental preparation. The opportunity to clear your mind will allow you to focus on creating winner strategies and formulas. It will also inspire a higher level of confidence and self esteem; ensuring you enter any competition in the right frame of mind. Just as importantly the float tank can provide an athlete with a space to unwind, analyse their performance and relax their muscles. A warm tank of water which makes you weightless will allow the aches and pains of the sport to fade away and can be the best possible way to start healing. This will ensure you are ready for peak performance again quicker than without this type of treatment. It is possible for your body to feel immediate relief from the pain as the pressure on your joints is immediately alleviated when you enter the water.

- Consciousness

The float tank was originally conceived to provide you with the opportunity to leave your own physical body and connect to other beings which either exist on a higher spiritual level or on the astral plane. While it is difficult to confirm how effective this part of the process is, there are many people who have experienced a temporary loss of consciousness and entered into a meditative state. It is when in this state that people are best able to see themselves and evaluate their capabilities and limits.

The time and space to enter into a state of higher consciousness also allows you to explore the world around you, your interaction with it and how it can be improved, both for your own benefit and for others. Entering a state of higher consciousness does not mean attempting to contact other life forms or even understand the meaning of life. What it does allow you to do is ascertain your place in the order of things and how your efforts can be used to improve life; both for yourself and for others around you. You may not reach this elevated state of enlightenment on your first attempt in the float tank but there are many of people who have experienced this after repeated visits to the float tank.

- Circulation

As the pressure is taken off your body, its internal organs and infrastructure can operate at peak capacity; your heart is able to pump more blood and oxygen around your body and your circulation will improve as there is little resistance to the blood flow. Although your body is better able to operate at peak capacity, it will not actually need to work as hard as normal. This will lower your blood pressure, reduce your heart rate and even lower your consumption of oxygen.

- Brain Waves

You should already be aware that the brain can start to shift from beta wave to theta waves, similar to the ones which go through your brain prior to falling asleep. What a float tank can also do is improve the co-ordination between the two sides of your brain. This can improve your mental clarity, co-ordination and increase your creativeness and problem solving skills.

Whatever your personal experience in a float tank you are certain to feel better for the time you have spent inside it. It will invigorate you, improve your health and inspire you to achieve more than you previously thought possible. Although scientists are still trying to understand the exact reasons why the float tank has such potential benefits, those who have used it can testify to the benefits they have felt and continue to feel.

SENSORY INTELLIGENCE

Soaking in a sensory deprivation tank is said to help improve your sensory intelligence. This is a relatively new field of study which looks at the ways you can change the way you think and act. It is intended to guide you into rethinking the way you approach work, life and how you learn. It is believed to be a good compliment to float tank treatment and can help to emphasize the benefits.

There are three main areas which are focused upon when dealing with sensory intelligence:

1. Senses on Call

Call centres are a fact of life and an essential part of many businesses. It is the first line of real contact between a customer and the business. Unfortunately the standard approach is geared at keeping the staff numbers up. This often results in poor quality staff and a high rate of turnover.

2. Senses at work

Hectic working environments have led to many employees failing to connect in their workplace and high levels of dissatisfaction is seen as normal and even acceptable. However, this can lead to high levels of staff turnover and low rats of productivity as staff are not engaged or happy at work.

3. Education

Children and their education are vitally important and yet it is a challenging and rapidly changing environment. The information which was relevant just ten years ago has very little effect on today's average child. As such, people need to learn to relate to the young people of today and ensure they have the skills necessary to achieve anything they want in life.

These points may seem far removed from the idea of sensory deprivation or float tans but they actually illustrate why it is so important to take the time out of your busy schedule to step back and take stock of your personal life and the wider world. Any parent can benefit from time in a float tank as they will realise what is actually important to them and the world around them. This will ensure they are able to offer the right level of assistance and direction which is so important to a child. They will also empower them as well as illustrating the importance of embracing new ideas.

Equally, the float tank can help bosses and world leaders to understand the principles which are important to their businesses and their employees. The float tank can raise the level of conscious awareness of others to ensure that the world becomes a fairer, happier place. This may seem like a bold claim, but any technique which forces you to evaluate your own sense of purpose and the welfare of those around you is a useful tool which can make the world a better place. Whilst there may still be debate on how effective the float tank is at helping people to attain higher levels of spirituality, there is no doubt that it does help people become more relaxed and focused; in much the same way as meditation can. Of course, meditation requires years of practice whilst sinking into a float tank will take you very little effort and assist you in reaching a meditative state.

Obviously improving the world for others is a noble goal and not the usual one that people start with when looking to try sensory deprivation for the first time. There are many reasons why you might wish to experience the reduction or elimination of your senses for a short period:

- Curiosity

One of the most powerful reasons to try anything is curiosity. If you have read this book and are thinking about trying you are already curious; if you do not follow through on this curiosity then it is likely to be one of those things that you will always end up regretting not trying. If the opportunity is there and affordable then there is little to stop you!

- Gift

If someone you know has tried the float tank or has read about it and decided it might be something that you would either be interested in or benefit from then you may find yourself being given a session. Just as with curiosity, this is an opportunity which is too good to pass up. All you need to do is attend with an open mind; you may be surprised by the benefits and the experience!

- Enlightenment

Those who have been to several sessions will report that they find it easier to unwind and see images, whether lights or pictures. It is believed that this is the freeing of the subconscious mind and it will enable you to be more creative as well as to reach an enlightened state such as many religious and notable people in the past have done through meditation. Enlightenment is, in reality, simply a state of mind which allows you to see and understand the importance of things within the order of the universe. This will allow you to see how small many issues really are and how you can deal with them or even ignore them.

- Pain relief

As this book has already covered, the float tank can offer instant pain relief for any joint sprains or muscle aches. This is because you are effectively weightless and all pressure is instantly removed from the area. Without pressure on it the joint or muscle is free to start healing, without risk of damage by adding significant pressure in the wrong direction.

- Stress relief

This book has also mentioned the abilities of a float tank to reduce the amount of stress you are under and how a period of reflection can help to reduce your stress levels and help you to evaluate the way forward. The emphasis is on focusing on the real issues and not getting stressed about the smaller matters; especially if they are beyond your control.

- Health Benefits

Sensory deprivation may also be something you are looking at as you have heard there is a range of health benefits, some of these may directly affect your health whilst others are simply to ensure you stay healthy:

- Magnesium

This is an essential metal which your body needs; it works to improve your circulation, increase your ability to absorb insulin, regulate electrolytes and, it can even reduce any muscle pain. Many people are actually deficient in Magnesium, but a stint in a float tank, with a vast amount of magnesium filled Epsom salts, will ensure your body has all the magnesium it needs.

- Creativity

As your brain slowly clears the hum of normal noise it becomes free to focus on any specific projects or aims you have. Your creativity can increase many times other as you allow your brain to focus on specific issues and find a range of solutions that had not previously occurred to you.

- Performance

Research shows that athletes and musicians can benefit massively from the use of float tans. Their attention levels rise and their visual – motor coordination improves as well as concentration levels.

- Hallucinations

This may seem like a peculiar benefit but it has been suggested that hallucinations help to free the mind and allow it to evaluate the options available. A float tank is the best way to experience hallucinations without needing to take illegal drugs or risking any harm to your body. Of course, it is not guaranteed to happen, but if you are curious about hallucinations, this is one of the best ways to try it safely.

- Disorders

There are a range of disorders which have been shown to be aided in either their treatment or in managing them by the use of a sensory deprivation tank; these include:

- Arthritis

- Migraines

- Insomnia

- Fibromyalgia – a degenerative disease.

- Improved Sleep

An additional benefit of session in a float tank has been shown to be an improved level of sleep; if you are struggling to get to sleep or sleep properly for any reason then the float tank can relax you sufficiently to ensure you experience the best night's sleep in a long time!

- Weight Loss

If you are trying to lose weight and struggling you may have heard that the float tank can assist with your aim. It will assist you to focus your mind on your objective and to see the right path to achieving it. This has been shown to be an effective way of starting and applying a weight loss technique. In fact clinical trials have proved the effectiveness of having just one sensory deprivation experience.

The list of reasons to try a float tank, combined with the range of reasons as to why it is a good idea should have you looking at where your closest float tank is and when you can go; to start experiencing these benefits.

THEORIES REGARDING THE BENEFITS

The sensory deprivation tank has been shown to offer a range of health benefits, many if these are backed up through comprehensive research and even clinical studies. However, there still remains a mystery regarding why this treatment method is so effective. There have been several theories put forwards as to why this is the case:

Gravity

Or, rather, the lack of gravity. It has been suggested that this lack of gravity is responsible for the remarkable range of benefits which can be gained from regular sessions in a float tank. The theory is that the brain can take a break from constantly orientating and adjusting the body as well as responding to countless number of stimuli. In everyday life the brain is constantly working, whether calculating which direction to move in, the best strategy to win a game or even engaging in a conversation. The float tank eliminates the need for the brain to do anything other than the most basic functions, the ones which are relatively autonomous, such as breathing of keeping your heart beating.

This theory is held up by research which suggests that ninety percent of the activity in the nervous system is connected with the pull of gravity on your body and the brain has to constantly recalibrate to allow for gravity, orientation and the right amount of force to ensure we move comfortably and fluidly. In effect, every movement of your muscles affects the balance of your body and requires more calculations by your brain. Floating on your back provides the maximum possible support to your body and alleviates the effects of gravity. This almost complete release from gravity not only frees the brain, it allows your body to heal, improve its circulation and for you to feel much smaller sensations than you would normally.

The Brain's Waves

Modern research is teaming the vast amount of knowledge regarding the human body from both the top Western research labs and the ancient medicinal and meditative arts; such as those taught by the Dhali Lama. The comparison of these techniques has shown that the brain waves in monks who enter deep meditative states, after years of practice are similar to those experienced by anyone in a float tank; whether their first time or one hundredth time! The brain switches from Beta waves to theta.

It is then reasonable to assume that the participation in a float tank session will give you access to the same meditative state as a monk who will have been practicing the technique for years. This means that float tanks really are a short cut to enlightenment!

Two Sides

The brain is designed as two halves; the left side and the right side are only connected by a thick bundle of nerves. Each side has been shown to have its own conscious thoughts and its own memories; the left side is known to control the right side of the body whilst the right brain controls the left side. Research shows that the two sides of the brain work in different ways and control different types of emotional states.

The right side controls the processing of non-verbal information in a non-linear timeless manner. It is associated with the moments when you have sudden clarity on a particular subject.

The left hand brain works in the opposite manner; it views all information logically and analytically, orientated in the specific time.

Most people have dominance in the left side of their brain, limiting their ability to be spontaneous and ensuring they take a logical and sensible approach to most issues. However, floating in a tank has been shown to help balance the sides of the brain. The right side becomes equal or dominant and allows your creative side to shine through. This is why you will feel more confident, capable and creative after a session in the float tank.

The Physiological Brain

It has been suggested that the brain actually consists of three brains which effectively sit on top of each other and are actually levels; each level corresponds to an evolutionary event in human history. This theory continues that each of the brains has its own memories, conscious and problem solving abilities. However, the brains are not very good at communicating with each other and this is a fundamental flaw in the human make-up. The three sections are:

- The reptile Brain – this is the oldest part of the brain and is a combination of the spinal cord, the brain stem and an area known as the midbrain. This is the part of the brain which covers basic functions such as reproduction and self-preservation. It is this part of the brain which alerts us to new things.

- Paleomammalian Brian – this part of your brain controls your emotional response and regulates body functions. It handles the day to day essentials such as hunger and thirst as well as sexual urges. In effect, it is the mood controlling part of your brain.

- Neocortex – this part handles cognitive function, including memory, intellect and judgment. It controls all voluntary movements and actions, (as opposed to sub conscious ones).

Research suggests that floating in a sensory deprivation tank allows the three brains to communicate far more effectively with each other than normal. This can lead to a clearer understanding of yourself and the world around you.

Biochemical

Chemicals are an essential part of your make-up, they provide a link between the physical and the non-physical; they make it possible to use your mind over matter! It is these neurochemicals that control your sexual arousal and your ability to feel either old or young. These chemicals also help to define your immune system. A lack of them can lead to a weak immune system. In fact, the level of these chemicals defines your emotional state and your ability to feel love, sadness, or passion.

This is particularly demonstrated by the presence of stress, when you are stressed your body will have elevated levels of cortisol and adrenaline. Floating has been linked to a reduction in these chemicals as your mind calms the neurochemicals lower the levels of cortisol and adrenaline, reducing your stress. In effect, your mood can control your body's reaction and your mood can be relaxed by the float tank.

The same principle applies to your entire range of emotional responses. Current research shows that regular use of a float tank can alter your brain chemistry in a positive way and help to regulate your mood, your behaviour and, most importantly, the strength of your immune system.

Homeostasis

Homeostasis is the interaction of all the different parts of the physical and emotional parts of the body in perfect harmony. Walter B. Cannon was a scientist he proposed the idea that the body has a finely tuned self-monitoring and self-regulating system which is working all the time to ensure the body achieves the perfect balance. Of course, this is a challenging concept as the perfect balance will be constantly affected by a wide array of outside forces. Homeostasis is not a fixed condition but rather a relative position dependent upon the demands and influences which surround you at any given time.

The float tank actually illustrates this point exceptionally well. It is not possible to be in the tank without it having an effect on your body, but likewise, the tank will have an effect on your mind, this will affect the way your body reacts and its current status. So the tank affects both the mind and the body, creating a shift in homeostasis!

The reason why the tank is so good for the body is that it once the shift in homeostasis has occurred, it becomes static; homeostasis is, temporarily, a fixed status. This is virtually impossible in the world outside of the tank where there are constant demands and pressures causing the homeostasis to need to change. It therefore follows that when your body is in the tank and a fixed homeostasis has been found, the body is actually free to apply all its resources to healing you or improving your spirituality.

Biofeedback

Research into brainwaves started as long ago as the 1960's. In the first instance scientists were studying the brain waves of animals. However, they quickly graduated to trying the sensors on themselves to see what the output was from their own brains. It took very little tile for them to realise that the output from a human brain, which is supposedly beyond our control, was actually controllable. The scientists could massively increase the amount of alpha waves emitting from their brains at will.

As the research continued it became apparent that it was actually possible to feed back a small specific signal. This signal was accepted by the brain and would be used to create a specific response; such as lowering the skin temperature or speeding up your heart beat. In fact, the research showed that it was possible to control ne specific neuron, if we wanted to. The human body is far more complicated and sophisticated than many people credit it to be!

This is possible simply because the scientists can feed back specific responses to the brain which will make it act in a certain way. However, it is possible to learn to control each of these minute body functions through this process. It is also possible to develop a much better control of all your organs, muscles and nerves through focusing your concentration and brain power on specific parts of your body. The float tank makes this more than just possible; it creates the perfect scenario to make it a reality. With the day to day clutter gone, your brain will be able to hear the smaller signals which are usually ignored. It can then specify what needs to be done and you will gain specific control over even the smallest of your body parts! Of course, this process takes practice and more than one session but the results are outstanding considering the human body is doing all the work!

TIPS TO HELP YOU RELAX AND PREPARE FOR THE FLOAT TANK

It is perfectly possible to simply turn up and jump straight into a float tank. However, as many people how have used one of these before will testify, you will get much more from your experience if you arrive prepared. To ensure you have the best possible experience you will find the following tips and guidelines useful:

- Eating and drinking

You are advised not to eat just before you go into the tank. If you do your stomach will still be digesting the food whilst you are floating. With no other distractions inside the tank you may be surprised at just how loud your digestive system can be! It may not ruin your experience but it will make it more difficult for you to settle and clear your mind. Ideally you should have your last food an hour or two before you enter the tank. Equally you should drink nothing for the two hours before your session. This will ensure you are able to empty your bladder just before entering the tank and you will not need to go again whilst you are in the tank; there is little which can be as annoying as having to come out of the tank half way through as needing to urinate. It is guaranteed to ruin your meditation zone!

It is worth noting that people generally recommend abstaining from any caffeine for at least twenty four hours before your float session; it will not help your brain clear and settle if you still have a stimulant in your body!

- The Towel

It is essential to check what towels, if any, are supplied at your chosen facility. You will need a towel to wrap around you as you come out of the tank; this one can also be used to wipe the majority of the salt off before you use the shower. You will, of course, need a towel for after your shower, when you are all clean and fresh.

Your towel that is to be used to wipe the salt off when you first emerge from the tank, should always be positioned near enough to the tank that you can access it from inside the tank without needing to shift position too much. If there is a towel hook inside the tank this is even better. The water you float in has a large amount of Epsom salts in; this will sting if it is accidentally dropped into your eye. It will not do any permanent damage but it will become uncomfortable and may make it difficult for you to concentrate on your session. Water usually goes into your eye when you move one of your arms around and it goes across your face. Having the towel easily accessible will allow you to quickly wipe away any excess salt and minimize any inconvenience.

- Time

As mentioned, the first time you have this treatment it will seem very peculiar and you may struggle to get comfortable. Whilst settling your mind as well as your body you may find yourself focusing on how long you have been in the tank or how long you have left. This is not something you should be thinking about; you are trying to clear your mind and thinking about the time is not going to help this.

The centre will ensure you know when your time is up, either by banging on the tank or via an underwater speaker which plays a short tune. This allows you a few minutes to adjust from your altered state of consciousness before you actually get out. It is possible to get the centre to play music for you for the first half or for the first and last five minutes.

- Breathing

You may be surprised at just how loud your breathing is once you are closed into the tank. However, this is actually a good thing! The loudness of your breathing provides a reassuring focal point. You should focus on your breathing and gradually slow your breathing down. This will help your mind to relax and your brain to stop thinking about anything else; it will empty itself of any other thoughts and help you to get into the right zone.

- Counting

If you are struggling with relaxing into what feels very much like an alien environment then one of the best methods you can try is simple counting. Just as with your breathing your focus will be on the counting and your brain will realise there is nothing else to do at the moment; this will ensure it relaxes and allows you to absorb your surroundings and make the most of the time you have in the tank.

- Sessions

Your first session should be at least one and a half hours long. It can be longer if you like but having a shorter session may make it difficult for you to get into the zone and experience the best possible results.

An hour and a half may seem like a long time but it will go past exceptionally quickly, there is also nothing stopping you getting out early or coming out for a few minutes in order to take a break. The more often you have float tank sessions the easier it will be for you to relax and 'get into the zone'; it will undoubtedly be more and more beneficial.

- Expectations

The experience of floating is different for every person. Even if you have been fifty times before it will not necessarily be the same as the time before. The best advice is to go with no expectations. Simply do your best to relax and let events take their course naturally. You cannot force your mind to focus on a particular issue as you will not be relaxing or disconnecting from the rest of the world; you will simply be mulling over one idea or principle whilst laid in a bath of warm water. In fact, focusing on an issue is likely to ensure you do not get the most out of your session.

You may not finish the session with the solution to all your problems but you will feel relaxed and more complete than you have done in a long time.

- Cuts

If you are unfortunate enough to have any cuts or open wounds on your body it is essential that they are covered with a waterproof plaster. This will ensure that the salt water does not touch your wound. If it does your nerves endings will do more than tingle, they will scream and you will definitely not gain a relaxing or enlightening experience!

- Pillow & Earplugs

Most places will supply new earplugs for you to use and an inflatable pillow. The choice of whether to use them or not is yours and is a matter of personal preference. Some people prefer to use a pillow to support their head and help them relax, others feel it is better not to have any kind of head support or earplugs and keep the experience as natural as possible. It is best to take one, if offered and try it both ways. If the centre does not offer a pillow you may wish to bring your own.

- Chlorine

It is very important that the water is filtered and kept clean for your safety. Some centres use UV and hydrogen peroxide, whilst others use chlorine. If the smell of chlorine bothers you then it is best to choose a different centre which uses an alternative to chlorine; this will help to ensure you relax as your sense of smell is not being assaulted the entire time!

- Extension

Many people feel like they are in a stupor, a world of their own when they exit from the tank. Their own actions seem slower, they feel exceptionally calm and everything around them seems to be in full colour HD compared to the normal black and white. Instead of rushing back to your normal life, enjoy the experience and assimilate what you have learned about yourself and the world around you. The best way to do this is to enjoy a cup of herbal tea, not coffee as this will stimulate your mind and body too quickly. Then simply relax for a short while, perhaps log your feelings to aid in the future.

- Meditation

It has been said that you can achieve the same depth of meditation after an hour in a float tank as many spiritual people achieve after years of studying and meditating daily. This allows you to experience things that the average person should not actually be able to achieve within their own busy schedule.

It can be even more beneficial if you either read up on meditation techniques or practice a few basic techniques prior to your appointment. This will ensure you can quickly relax and find an altered state of mind, allowing you to get the best possible experience.

Entering with the right preparation will ensure you get the most from your time in the tank; it will also allow you to arrive relaxed and prepared; this will help you to settle into one of the most unique experiences you will ever have.

CONCLUSION

Sensory deprivation has come a long way since its initial inception in the 1960's. It was once the brainchild of a well meaning scientist who got carried away with adding drugs to the mix and attempting to observe the effects. Despite this start the benefits were recognised and the float tank was born, refined and improved. Unfortunately the AIDs scare of the 1980's affected the popularity of the float tank as people were scared that they would catch HIV or AIDs from the water. It was also associated with interrogation techniques and this left many people not wanting to be connected with the trend. However, instead of disappearing the trend simply paused and reappeared twenty five years later; it is now rapidly growing in popularity and businesses are appearing around the world as more and more people become hooked on the idea and the experience.

Sensory deprivation offers an impressive range of benefits, ranging from health benefits to the relief of anxiety and even the ability to reach a higher state of consciousness. However, despite the evidence which backs up these claims there are surprisingly little scientific reasons as to why the float tank has such a positive effect on the human body. Research is continuing but at present there can be little doubt as to the benefits which can be had by spending a small amount of time in one of these tanks.

There are many theories as to why spending time in a sensory deprivation tank has some many benefits to the mind and body; however, all of the ones discussed in this book are simply theories and suppositions. Each one of them has potential and offers a reasonable explanation; the truth is that all of them may well be relevant to the real reason the float tank has become such a success and why it has such a positive effect on the body. It is certainly true that being allowed to have some downtime, away from the stresses and the strains of the world has always been seen as a good thing. The usual resort was a good book, a long walk or a deep tissue massage. The float tank takes this one stage further and provides you with the opportunity to escape from yourself as well as the world around you. Almost everyone will be able to see the appeal in this idea; an opportunity to shut down completely will recharge your batteries. What the theories do not foresee is the general feeling of well being which you acquire after each session and the addictive nature of the treatment.

The concept of an empty mind is almost impossible to fathom unless you have actually experienced it. No matter how quiet your mind appears to be there are always hundreds of questions popping up, your mind looks for solutions; the sheer number of things going round inside your mind can be seen when you first settle into a float tank and attempt to enter your mind. The first time you ever experience this opportunity to achieve an empty mind you will struggle to clear all the thoughts running through your head.

The float tank offers an acceptable and affordable way to relieve stress, anxiety and achieve a state of true relaxation without the need to resort to any medical answer or drugs; prescription or otherwise. It has also been shown to help reduce the effects of pain and assist you to achieve a higher state of consciousness where you will be able to see what truly matters and focus on the bigger picture. All of these topics have been covered by this book and, by now, you should have a good understanding of all the principles and procedures involved in using a float tank. The essential tips will ensure you prepare properly for your experience and the guide to your float tank session will ensure you know what to expect before you get there. Providing you undertake your homework and choose a facility which has a high level of hygiene and professionalism you will have an enjoyable and rewarding experience.

Before it is possible to appreciate the range of effects that this type of treatment can have it is essential to understand the causes of sensory overload in the modern world. This book delves into the variety of sensory overload which can affect anyone; there are several ways of dealing with sensory overload, although, regular sessions in a float tank offers the greatest benefit. The book also touches on the idea of sensory intelligence and how this can relate to sensory deprivation. There are no known negative side effects of regular sessions in a float tank unless you spend an extended amount of time in one and indulge in substances which are not recommended; particularly drugs. The likely outcome of this is that you will experience hallucinations, although these are not harmful in themselves. The float tank offers the ultimate opportunity to explore yourself and the world around you; if you haven't experienced it yet then perhaps it is time you booked your appointment!

Made in the USA
Columbia, SC
09 April 2021